DIY Essential Oils
How To Make Your Own Essential Oils

Table of content

Introduction

There you are, browsing the department store, looking at all of the shelves full of different essential oils. Or perhaps you prefer to take your shopping to the online realm, and you find that your minutes are spent on Amazon or another website looking at page after page of essential oils, just waiting for you to click on that 'order' button.

But, you still have your standards, and you know what you want with your essential oils. It doesn't matter what you want to do with them, whether you are using them for aroma therapy, you are using them in different teas or other remedies that you want to make yourself, or if you are going to use them for topical purposes only.

No matter what your reason is, you need to find the best of the best in the essential oil realm, and you want to be absolutely certain the oils you choose are the oils for you.

"I have never gone through the process of making oils... is there a way I can do it myself?"

"I want to make my own oils and save time and money in the long run... is it that hard to do?"

"I want to make my own oils, but I've never done it before, and I don't want to mess it up."

If you have ever felt any of these thoughts, or if you have ever had your hesitations about making your own essential oils, set them aside. You are about to discover everything you need to know about making your own essential oils, and how you can keep yourself well supplied with what you have on hand.

This book is going to show you the secrets behind essential oils, and just what you need to do to take them from something you buy in a little bottle to something you can make yourself, in as big or as little amounts as you wish.

Let this book change the way you do your oils, and discover how easy it is to make your own, no matter what you want to do with them. This book is going to open the door for you, showing you that you can make any kind of essential oil that you want, whenever you want, wherever you are.

Chapter 1 – Getting Started: A Method To Your Madness

I know there is a lot of excitement when you are starting any new hobby, and making your own essential oils is at the top of the list for many people. There's so much more satisfaction out of a product when you do a lot of the work yourself, and essential oils can be used in such a diverse amount of ways, there's no telling how many ways you can be self-sufficient in this realm.

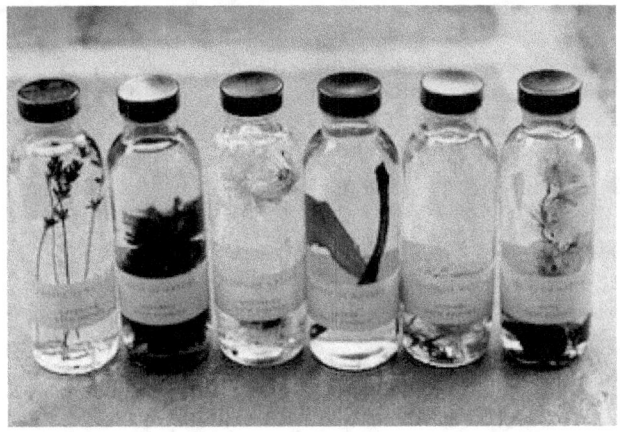

Before you jump in with a press and some fruit, however, we need to take a few minutes and discuss the different ways you can obtain your oils. Thankfully, essentials are easy to come by, so you aren't going to have an issue at all in getting the oil you want.

The yin yang of steams and presses

The two many methods by which people get essential oils are through either steaming the matter, or pressing the matter. There are pros and cons to both, and in the chapters to come, we are going to closely examine both methods and you can choose for yourself the method you wish to use in your extraction.

I personally find that I like using both methods for different kinds of oils, so don't be afraid to embrace what you feel is more you... there's no right or wrong method between these two, they are simply different.

With that in mind, let's take a look at them, and how they are different from each other.

The press method:

This method of extraction really is as easy as it sounds. Basically, you will use the matter of your choice, whether this is herbs, fruit, the rinds of fruit, or any combination in between, and you will mechanically press the matter until you get the oils.

Odds are you have done this by accident at some point in your life, or even done so when you were playing around as a child. Either way, this is a very basic and easy method to use when you want to get oils quickly.

Although it is an efficient way to get the oils, it is important to keep in mind that these oils you will get out of the matter aren't officially essential oils. But, don't let that get you down or stop you, because you not only can use the oils you get just the same as essential oils, odds are you won't even be able to tell the difference between the two.

The steam method

In a nutshell, the other way you can get essential oils is through steaming. There are several different processes within this category that you can use to get the oils, and I recommend that you try them all and find which one works for you.

Keep in mind when you steam the matter to get the oils, you are going to be working with hot items, and you can get burned. Make sure you keep everything out of reach of children, and that you are careful yourself as you work through the process.

Take your time, there is no rush, and be sure you pay attention to detail. The more you practice at it, the easier it is going to get.

So let's take a look at the different methods used within this steam method:

Water alone

You will use a pot of boiling water to get the oils you are after. This is basic, simple, and can be done in little time. You do have to keep a close eye on the matter as it boils, but overall this is the easiest method to use when you are getting the oils.

Steam alone

If you have ever steamed vegetables than you already have a good idea of how to go about this method. There are more things you need to be careful of, but it is a fast and easy way to get the oils out of the plants.

Water and steam combined

You may like one thing, you may like another, or you may be one of those people that doesn't like to choose when you can have both. If you like the steam method, and you like the water method, don't make yourself choose which one you want to do, do them both.

I will show you how you can get the oils you want out of the methods separately, then combine the methods to get oils in a fast and easy way. No matter how you want to do it, you are going to get your oils, so mess around with the methods and discover which one you want for yourself.

The result:

At the end of the day, there's really no right or wrong way to get the oils if you follow this steps, but there are going to be definite differences for you as the process goes on.

I don't want to tell you which ones are best and which ones aren't, because it really does come down to personal preference at one point or another. In the chapters to come, I am going to show you how you can make your own oils using any one of these methods, and you can try them all.

Discover which one you like, and use that as your go-to method.

Either way, have fun with it and love the process.

Chapter 2 – I'm Impressed: The Cold Press Oil Method

There are three different ways you can use water to get the oils out of the matter of choice, but the press method is very straight forward. In it, you will find that the way you get the oils is very step by step, and the results are predictable.

Let's take a look now at how you can do this method to get your oils, and the things you will need to make that happen.

Needed supplies:

Plant matter

Pestle

Extraction oil

Directions:

The way you execute the cold press method is just as simple as it sounds. You are going to literally press the oils out of the matter.

Keep in mind that you will need a lot of plant matter to get essential oils, so always plan on getting minimal amounts of oil no matter how many plants you put into your project.

Now, take your plant matter, and place it in your bowl. You can use a pestle and mortar as I prefer, or you can use a simply bowl, either way, make sure it isn't plastic, as this is going to cling to the oils.

Cover the plant matter with an extraction oil. I prefer to use jojoba oil, but you can use almond oil or fractionated coconut oil if you like. Let sit in the plant matter for two full days.

Keep an eye on it during this time, as you need to make sure the plants are covered in the oil. You may need to add a little more oil from time to time as the plant matter shifts and adjusts within the container.

After the 48 hours, use the pestle to crush the plant matter. Of course, you will need to move slowly to keep the oils in the bowl. The last thing you want to happen is having your oils fly around the room as you work.

Continue to deliberately press and stir, press and stir until you have all of the matter thoroughly crushed. Don't worry about how small the matter gets, you are going to strain the oil before use to remove any of the large pieces.

After you are satisfied with the oil, set it aside, and grab another glass bowl. Line this bowl with cheese cloth, and slowly pour your oil and plant matter blend into the cheese cloth. You need to move slowly as you go along to make sure you don't splash out any of the oils.

Gather up the ends of the cheese cloth next, and secure them together. Hang over the bowl for another 24 hours, until all of the oil has drained out of the plant matter into your bowl. I personally find it helpful to put on rubber gloves and squeeze the remaining oil out of the blend.

Once I have my strained oil in a dish, I transfer it into a dark glass bottle. Screw the lid on tightly before storing. Your oils will stay fresh for up to 6 months.

Chapter 3 – Sauna With A Purpose: Steam and Water Methods

While there are a lot of benefits to using the good old pestle and mortar, you are going to find that water and steam do hold their own in the grand scheme of things. Not only are you able to be more hands free while obtaining your oils, but you can fix it and forget it while the oils basically remove themselves from the plant matter.

The drawback of these methods as opposed to the cold pressed method is that you are going to have to wait longer to get the oils, but all in all, the amount of hands on time you spend in the kitchen isn't going to compare. So you can really pick and choose which method works better for you.

So, let's plunge onward into the water and steam methods.

Water alone:

Place your plant matter into your crock pot. Cover generously with water.

Turn crockpot on high, and keep an eye on the plant matter. I like to stir a few times, but this is not necessary if you are unable to stand there with it. Once the water starts to boil, turn the crockpot down to medium.

You want the plant matter to continue to boil in the crock, so keep an eye on it and make sure that the water continues to boil. Add water as necessary, and let the plants boil for up to eight hours.

After the eight hours, turn the crockpot off and uncover. Now you must let the water sit undisturbed for three to four days. Sometimes I even leave it up to a week, but if you need it sooner, go ahead and skim the water when you are ready.

You will see the oils collect at the top of the water. Use a spoon to scoop off the oils and set aside. Once all of the oil has been skimmed, discard the contents of the crock pot, and let the bowl of oils sit out for another twenty-four hours. The rest of the water will evaporate, and your oils are going to be left in the bowl.

Steaming method:

In steaming essential oils, you are going to be a lot more hands on than when you use the water method, but the method is faster in general as opposed to the water method alone.

Place your plant matter into your crock pot. Cover generously with water.

Turn crockpot on high, and keep an eye on the plant matter. I like to stir a few times, but this is not necessary if you are unable to stand there with it. Once the water starts to boil, turn the crockpot down to medium.

You want the plant matter to boil in the crock, so keep an eye on it and make sure that the water continues to boil.

Leave a glass in the center of the crock. This needs to be firm enough to not tip over in the water, but above the water line. You can place weight in the bottom of it to keep it in place if you like.

Make sure the lid can also close on the crock. As the water boils, the steam is going to gather in and over the glass. Let it continue to collect for a few hours.

Once the time has passed, remove the glass from the crockpot. Be careful as the glass and water inside are going to be very hot. Don't burn yourself or break the glass as you work. Set the glass aside and let sit for up to 2 days.

The water is going to evaporate, and the oil will be left behind.

I know this is a tedious method, but there are evaporators available if you want to speed up the process. The drawback is that they are expensive, but if you want to use steam method alone to collect your essential oils, you may want to look into that method as an option.

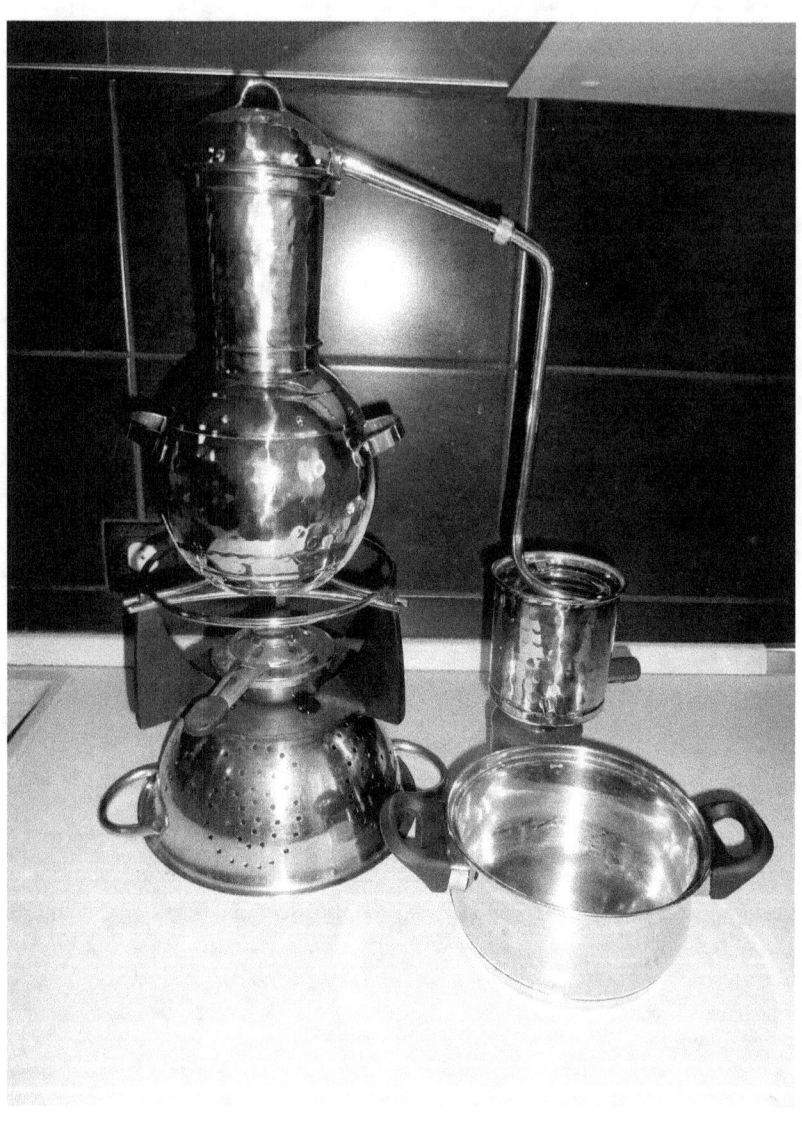

The steam and water method

The best way to combine the two methods for essential oil extraction is to do that very thing... you are going to take the best of both methods and combine them to get the result that you want.

Once again, you must place your plant matter into your crock pot. Cover generously with water.

Turn crockpot on high, and keep an eye on the plant matter. I like to stir a few times, but this is not necessary if you are unable to stand there with it. Once the water starts to boil, turn the crockpot down to medium.

You want the plant matter to boil in the crock, so keep an eye on it and make sure that the water continues to boil. Let the water boil over the plant matter for eight to ten hours, and when the time has passed, once again skim the water into another dish.

Now, instead of letting the dish sit, you are going to transfer the dish to another pot, and place this on the stove. Cover the pot with a lid so the steam doesn't all escape, and turn the burner on to high.

Keep an eye on the water, you don't want it to boil dry, but you do want it to boil for an hour or two, enough to boil off a lot of the excess water that is still in the oil. When you see that your water level is low, remove from the heat and set on the counter with the lid still on.

After a couple hours, remove the lid, and let the water mix continue to sit for a few more hours. The rest of the water will evaporate, and you will be left with the oil in the bottom of your pan.

No matter which method you decide to use, once the oil has cooled and the water has been removed, transfer the oil to a dark glass bottle with a lid. Secure the lid before storage, and your oils are going to stay nice for up to twelve months.

Chapter 4 – Stone Cold: Cold Pressed Recipes

I thought you would be eager to begin your own oils, so I have decided to include the directions for you to make ten different kinds, and I have included five in each method, so you can pick and choose as you please.

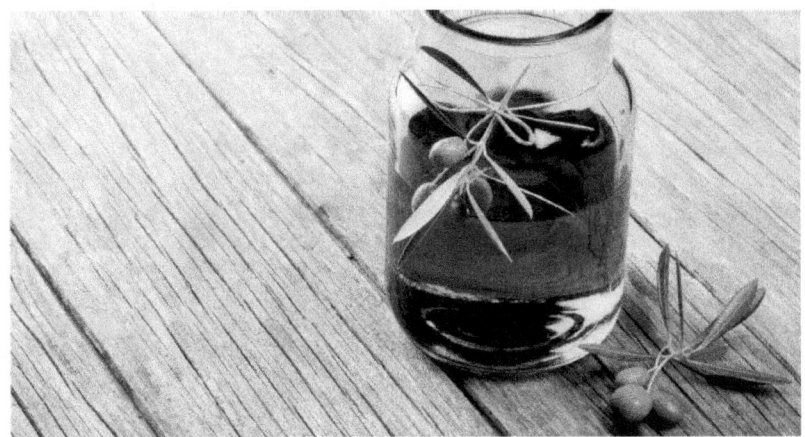

Here are the oils I love to press out by hand. Mix and match as you please, and discover how you like your blends. Remember that there's no wrong way to oil, so dive in with both hands and you will get what you are after!

The Caveman Blend

You will need:

1 large handful lemongrass

1 smaller handful lemon mint

1 cup jojoba oil (adjusted to your preference and needs)

Pestle and mortar

Follow the method directions found in chapter 2 to make these oils. Remember to take your time with the process and keep everything in the bowl as much as possible.

The Pioneer Blend

You will need:

1 large handful wheatgrass

1 smaller handful lilac petals

1 small handful rose petals

1 cup jojoba oil (adjusted to your preference and needs)

Pestle and mortar

Follow the method directions found in chapter 2 to make these oils. Remember to take your time with the process and keep everything in the bowl as much as possible.

Fresh Squeezed Citrus

You will need:

1 large handful lemon peels (some fruit left in is fine)

1 smaller handful orange peels (again, fruit left in is fine)

1 cup jojoba oil (adjusted to your preference and needs)

Pestle and mortar

Follow the method directions found in chapter 2 to make these oils. Remember to take your time with the process and keep everything in the bowl as much as possible.

The Minty Madness

You will need:

1 large handful peppermint

1 smaller handful spearmint

1 small handful mint leaves of your choice (or just plain mint)

1 cup jojoba oil (adjusted to your preference and needs)

Pestle and mortar

Follow the method directions found in chapter 2 to make these oils. Remember to take your time with the process and keep everything in the bowl as much as possible.

Everything You Need (And Nothing You Don't)

You will need:

1 large handful fresh basil

1 smaller handful lavender flowers

1 small handful wheatgrass

1 cup jojoba oil (adjusted to your preference and needs)

Pestle and mortar

Follow the method directions found in chapter 2 to make these oils. Remember to take your time with the process and keep everything in the bowl as much as possible.

Chapter 5 – Turning Up The Heat: Steam Method

Of course for every story there is two sides, and for every method, there is another method you would love to try out as well.

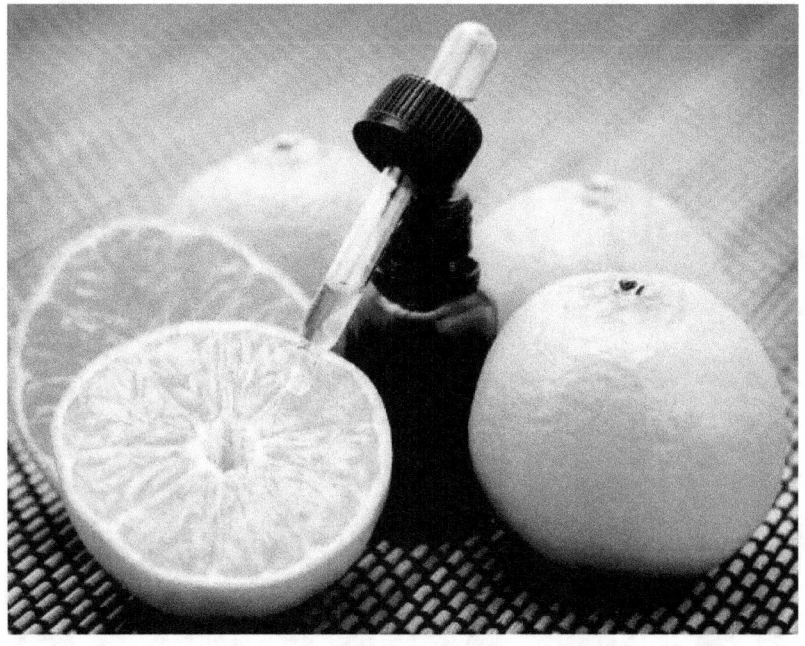

I promised you two different sets of recipes, and that is exactly what you are getting. These blends are designed for the steam method, but you can use them in the cold press method if you prefer.

And on the other side of that, you can use the cold pressed recipes in the steam method as well if that is what you want to do. Have fun with it and see what you come up with. The more you explore, the more incredible varieties you are going to discover!

The Steamy Sauna

You will need:

1 large rose petals

1 smaller sunflower petals

1 handful lilac petals

Enough water to cover the bottom of the pot, or to completely cover the plant matter, depending on your personal preference

Crock pot and bowl

Follow the method directions found in chapter 3 to make these oils. Remember to take your time with the process and keep everything in the bowl as much as possible.

The Sweet Dew

You will need:

1 large handful peppermint leaves

1 smaller handful cinnamon sticks

Enough water to cover the bottom of the pot, or to completely cover the plant matter, depending on your personal preference

Crock pot and bowl

Follow the method directions found in chapter 3 to make these oils. Remember to take your time with the process and keep everything in the bowl as much as possible.

Steamed Garden Blend

You will need:

1 large handful fresh parsley

1 smaller handful fresh basil

1 handful cilantro

1 small chopped piece of ginger

Enough water to cover the bottom of the pot, or to completely cover the plant matter, depending on your personal preference

Crock pot and bowl

Follow the method directions found in chapter 3 to make these oils. Remember to take your time with the process and keep everything in the bowl as much as possible.

Sugar and Spice is Everything Nice

You will need:

1 large handful cinnamon sticks

1 smaller handful chopped fresh ginger cubes

1 cup orange peels (fruit left on the pieces are fine)

Enough water to cover the bottom of the pot, or to completely cover the plant matter, depending on your personal preference

Crock pot and bowl

Follow the method directions found in chapter 3 to make these oils. Remember to take your time with the process and keep everything in the bowl as much as possible.

Perfection In A Blend

You will need:

1 large handful peppermint

1 smaller handful fresh lemon peels (pieces of fruit left on the peel are just fine)

1 small handful lavender petals

1 small handful rose petals

Enough water to cover the bottom of the pot, or to completely cover the plant matter, depending on your personal preference

Crock pot and bowl

Follow the method directions found in chapter 3 to make these oils. Remember to take your time with the process and keep everything in the bowl as much as possible.

That's all you really need to do to make your own essential oils. As with anything, you can expect to run into some roadblocks as you work through this, but the more you keep at it, the easier it is going to be, and the more plants you will be able to get use out of.

There are, however, a few things you need to keep in mind, and I have included them here. I don't want you to stress about making your own oils, but there are a few things everyone who makes their own oils needs to know. These are more safety and general information tips so you know what to expect from your oils, and you know exactly what you can use the oils for.

While you will easily be able to make your own oils out of virtually any kind of plant, you have to keep in mind which plants are toxic. I never recommend you consume any of these oils.

You will have a lot of fun while you make your own oils, but you may not save money, because you aren't going to get very much oil out of the plants you use. This doesn't mean that you shouldn't make them yourself, but you do need to know what to expect out of the oils you use.

These are not as potent as the essential oils that you purchase in the store. They are extremely useful, but don't expect them to be exactly like the store oils.

As with any hobby you engage in, you need to know what to expect while you work. This is going to greatly increase the benefits you get from the oils you are using, and it is going to help you know which plants to choose when you are in the mood to make more oils.

Just remember, above all, have fun with it. Use this as a stress reliever, and you are going to both have a good time while you work, and enjoy the product you get when you are done. All in all, you are setting yourself up to get the best of both worlds, and nothing can compare to that.

So get out there and explore the different kinds of options you have available to you right in your own back yard, and you will never be without the plants you want to make any kind of oil you imagine.

Let the fun begin.

Conclusion

There you have it, everything you need to know to get yourself started in the essential oil kitchen, and to take your hobby from something you are trying out to something you want to do on a regular basis.

I know there is a lot of excitement when you are starting any new hobby, but it is important that you take the time to do it right, and that you don't rush through anything and make a mistake because of it. There are so many essential oils you will be able to make, you can slow down and enjoy the journey with them.

The more you work at it, the better it is going to become, and the more experienced you are going to be with your essential oils. I want this book to take you from the very beginning, and build up the confidence you need to take this hobby to the next level, no matter how much experience you have in this.

Get your supplies, get your bottles, and get the fruit and herbs you need to make your own oils, and in no time at all you are going to be on top of the world, knowing that you are getting exactly what you are after in the process. No more wondering if what you have is pure, no more wondering if you are getting cheated or swindled, no more hoping you are getting the oils you pay for.

With this book, you can see the process for yourself, and you can get exactly what you want with your oils. There's no guesswork, no games, and no dealing with companies you don't trust.

This book is going to put you in total control of the essential oils you have in your cupboard, and it is going to make it easy for you to get more any time you need them. There's not going to be any more stress of them not having what you need in stock, there's not going to be any more wondering if you can even find the oil that you want, and there's going to be no more shipping times to wait for.

This book is going to show you exactly what you need to take your hobby from an idea to the next level. You are going to find everything you need right here, and in no time you will be able to make anything you need any time you want it.

Let me show you just how easy it is to get what you want, when you want it, and how you can customize, perfect, and obtain exactly what you are looking for in incredibly little time. This book is going to change the way you do essential oils, and it is going to change the way you craft, period.

So what are you waiting for? You have everything you need right here, so jump in there and make those oils. You are going to be so very glad you did.

www.ingramcontent.com/pod-product-compliance
Lightning Source LLC
Chambersburg PA
CBHW061946280526
45787CB00004B/1742